Tea

Type _____ **Region** _____

Date _____

I0424769

Appearance		☆ ☆ ☆ ☆ ☆
Aroma		☆ ☆ ☆ ☆ ☆
Body		☆ ☆ ☆ ☆ ☆
Taste		☆ ☆ ☆ ☆ ☆
Finish		☆ ☆ ☆ ☆ ☆

Tasting Notes	Temp & Brew time

Thoughts

Ratings ☆ ☆ ☆ ☆ ☆

Tea

Type _____ Region _____

Date _____

Appearance		☆ ☆ ☆ ☆ ☆
Aroma		☆ ☆ ☆ ☆ ☆
Body		☆ ☆ ☆ ☆ ☆
Taste		☆ ☆ ☆ ☆ ☆
Finish		☆ ☆ ☆ ☆ ☆

Tasting Notes	Temp & Brew time

Thoughts

Ratings ☆ ☆ ☆ ☆ ☆

Tea _____

Type _____ Region _____

Date _____

Appearance		☆ ☆ ☆ ☆ ☆
Aroma		☆ ☆ ☆ ☆ ☆
Body		☆ ☆ ☆ ☆ ☆
Taste		☆ ☆ ☆ ☆ ☆
Finish		☆ ☆ ☆ ☆ ☆

Tasting Notes	Temp & Brew time

Thoughts

Ratings ☆ ☆ ☆ ☆ ☆

Tea

Type _____ Region _____

Date _____

Appearance		☆ ☆ ☆ ☆ ☆
Aroma		☆ ☆ ☆ ☆ ☆
Body		☆ ☆ ☆ ☆ ☆
Taste		☆ ☆ ☆ ☆ ☆
Finish		☆ ☆ ☆ ☆ ☆

Tasting Notes	Temp & Brew time

Thoughts

Ratings ☆ ☆ ☆ ☆ ☆

Tea

Type _____ **Region** _____

Date _____

Appearance		☆ ☆ ☆ ☆ ☆
Aroma		☆ ☆ ☆ ☆ ☆
Body		☆ ☆ ☆ ☆ ☆
Taste		☆ ☆ ☆ ☆ ☆
Finish		☆ ☆ ☆ ☆ ☆

Tasting Notes	Temp & Brew time

Thoughts

Ratings ☆ ☆ ☆ ☆ ☆

Tea _____

Type _____ Region _____

Date _____

Appearance		☆ ☆ ☆ ☆ ☆
Aroma		☆ ☆ ☆ ☆ ☆
Body		☆ ☆ ☆ ☆ ☆
Taste		☆ ☆ ☆ ☆ ☆
Finish		☆ ☆ ☆ ☆ ☆

Tasting Notes	Temp & Brew time

Thoughts

Ratings ☆ ☆ ☆ ☆ ☆

Tea

Type _____ **Region** _____

Date _____

Appearance		☆ ☆ ☆ ☆ ☆
Aroma		☆ ☆ ☆ ☆ ☆
Body		☆ ☆ ☆ ☆ ☆
Taste		☆ ☆ ☆ ☆ ☆
Finish		☆ ☆ ☆ ☆ ☆

Tasting Notes	Temp & Brew time

Thoughts

Ratings ☆ ☆ ☆ ☆ ☆

Tea

Type _____ **Region** _____

Date _____

Appearance		☆ ☆ ☆ ☆ ☆
Aroma		☆ ☆ ☆ ☆ ☆
Body		☆ ☆ ☆ ☆ ☆
Taste		☆ ☆ ☆ ☆ ☆
Finish		☆ ☆ ☆ ☆ ☆

Tasting Notes	Temp & Brew time

Thoughts

Ratings ☆ ☆ ☆ ☆ ☆

Tea _____

Type _____ Region _____

Date _____

Appearance		☆ ☆ ☆ ☆ ☆
Aroma		☆ ☆ ☆ ☆ ☆
Body		☆ ☆ ☆ ☆ ☆
Taste		☆ ☆ ☆ ☆ ☆
Finish		☆ ☆ ☆ ☆ ☆

Tasting Notes	Temp & Brew time

Thoughts

Ratings ☆ ☆ ☆ ☆ ☆

Tea

Type _____ Region _____

Date _____

Appearance		☆ ☆ ☆ ☆ ☆
Aroma		☆ ☆ ☆ ☆ ☆
Body		☆ ☆ ☆ ☆ ☆
Taste		☆ ☆ ☆ ☆ ☆
Finish		☆ ☆ ☆ ☆ ☆

Tasting Notes	Temp & Brew time

Thoughts

Ratings ☆ ☆ ☆ ☆ ☆

Tea

Tea _____

Type _____ Region _____

Date _____

Appearance		☆ ☆ ☆ ☆ ☆
Aroma		☆ ☆ ☆ ☆ ☆
Body		☆ ☆ ☆ ☆ ☆
Taste		☆ ☆ ☆ ☆ ☆
Finish		☆ ☆ ☆ ☆ ☆

Tasting Notes	Temp & Brew time

Thoughts

Ratings ☆ ☆ ☆ ☆ ☆

Tea

Type _____ Region _____

Date _____

Appearance		☆ ☆ ☆ ☆ ☆
Aroma		☆ ☆ ☆ ☆ ☆
Body		☆ ☆ ☆ ☆ ☆
Taste		☆ ☆ ☆ ☆ ☆
Finish		☆ ☆ ☆ ☆ ☆

Tasting Notes	Temp & Brew time

Thoughts

Ratings ☆ ☆ ☆ ☆ ☆

Tea _____

Type _____ Region _____

Date _____

Appearance		☆ ☆ ☆ ☆ ☆
Aroma		☆ ☆ ☆ ☆ ☆
Body		☆ ☆ ☆ ☆ ☆
Taste		☆ ☆ ☆ ☆ ☆
Finish		☆ ☆ ☆ ☆ ☆

Tasting Notes	Temp & Brew time

Thoughts

Ratings ☆ ☆ ☆ ☆ ☆

Tea

Type _____ Region _____

Date _____

Appearance		☆ ☆ ☆ ☆ ☆
Aroma		☆ ☆ ☆ ☆ ☆
Body		☆ ☆ ☆ ☆ ☆
Taste		☆ ☆ ☆ ☆ ☆
Finish		☆ ☆ ☆ ☆ ☆

Tasting Notes	Temp & Brew time

Thoughts

Ratings ☆ ☆ ☆ ☆ ☆

Tea _____

Type _____ Region _____

Date _____

Appearance		☆ ☆ ☆ ☆ ☆
Aroma		☆ ☆ ☆ ☆ ☆
Body		☆ ☆ ☆ ☆ ☆
Taste		☆ ☆ ☆ ☆ ☆
Finish		☆ ☆ ☆ ☆ ☆

Tasting Notes	Temp & Brew time

Thoughts

Ratings ☆ ☆ ☆ ☆ ☆

Tea

Type _____ Region _____

Date _____

Appearance		☆ ☆ ☆ ☆ ☆
Aroma		☆ ☆ ☆ ☆ ☆
Body		☆ ☆ ☆ ☆ ☆
Taste		☆ ☆ ☆ ☆ ☆
Finish		☆ ☆ ☆ ☆ ☆

Tasting Notes	Temp & Brew time

Thoughts

Ratings ☆ ☆ ☆ ☆ ☆

Tea _____

Type _____ Region _____

Date _____

Appearance		☆ ☆ ☆ ☆ ☆
Aroma		☆ ☆ ☆ ☆ ☆
Body		☆ ☆ ☆ ☆ ☆
Taste		☆ ☆ ☆ ☆ ☆
Finish		☆ ☆ ☆ ☆ ☆

Tasting Notes	Temp & Brew time

Thoughts

Ratings ☆ ☆ ☆ ☆ ☆

Tea

Type _____ Region _____

Date _____

Appearance		☆ ☆ ☆ ☆ ☆
Aroma		☆ ☆ ☆ ☆ ☆
Body		☆ ☆ ☆ ☆ ☆
Taste		☆ ☆ ☆ ☆ ☆
Finish		☆ ☆ ☆ ☆ ☆

Tasting Notes	Temp & Brew time

Thoughts

Ratings ☆ ☆ ☆ ☆ ☆

Tea

Type _____ **Region** _____

Date _____

Appearance		☆ ☆ ☆ ☆ ☆
Aroma		☆ ☆ ☆ ☆ ☆
Body		☆ ☆ ☆ ☆ ☆
Taste		☆ ☆ ☆ ☆ ☆
Finish		☆ ☆ ☆ ☆ ☆

Tasting Notes	Temp & Brew time

Thoughts

Ratings ☆ ☆ ☆ ☆ ☆

Tea

Type _____ Region _____

Date _____

Appearance		☆ ☆ ☆ ☆ ☆
Aroma		☆ ☆ ☆ ☆ ☆
Body		☆ ☆ ☆ ☆ ☆
Taste		☆ ☆ ☆ ☆ ☆
Finish		☆ ☆ ☆ ☆ ☆

Tasting Notes	Temp & Brew time

Thoughts

Ratings ☆ ☆ ☆ ☆ ☆

Tea

Type _____ Region _____

Date _____

		Rating
Appearance		☆ ☆ ☆ ☆ ☆
Aroma		☆ ☆ ☆ ☆ ☆
Body		☆ ☆ ☆ ☆ ☆
Taste		☆ ☆ ☆ ☆ ☆
Finish		☆ ☆ ☆ ☆ ☆

Tasting Notes	Temp & Brew time

Thoughts

Ratings ☆ ☆ ☆ ☆ ☆

Tea

Type _____ Region _____

Date _____

Appearance		☆ ☆ ☆ ☆ ☆
Aroma		☆ ☆ ☆ ☆ ☆
Body		☆ ☆ ☆ ☆ ☆
Taste		☆ ☆ ☆ ☆ ☆
Finish		☆ ☆ ☆ ☆ ☆

Tasting Notes	Temp & Brew time

Thoughts

Ratings ☆ ☆ ☆ ☆ ☆

Tea

Type _____ Region _____

Date _____

Appearance		☆ ☆ ☆ ☆ ☆
Aroma		☆ ☆ ☆ ☆ ☆
Body		☆ ☆ ☆ ☆ ☆
Taste		☆ ☆ ☆ ☆ ☆
Finish		☆ ☆ ☆ ☆ ☆

Tasting Notes	Temp & Brew time

Thoughts

Ratings ☆ ☆ ☆ ☆ ☆

Tea

Type _____ Region _____

Date _____

Appearance		☆ ☆ ☆ ☆ ☆
Aroma		☆ ☆ ☆ ☆ ☆
Body		☆ ☆ ☆ ☆ ☆
Taste		☆ ☆ ☆ ☆ ☆
Finish		☆ ☆ ☆ ☆ ☆

Tasting Notes	Temp & Brew time

Thoughts

Ratings ☆ ☆ ☆ ☆ ☆

Tea

Type _____ Region _____

Date _____

Appearance		☆ ☆ ☆ ☆ ☆
Aroma		☆ ☆ ☆ ☆ ☆
Body		☆ ☆ ☆ ☆ ☆
Taste		☆ ☆ ☆ ☆ ☆
Finish		☆ ☆ ☆ ☆ ☆

Tasting Notes	Temp & Brew time

Thoughts

Ratings ☆ ☆ ☆ ☆ ☆

Tea _____

Type _____ Region _____

Date _____

Appearance		☆ ☆ ☆ ☆ ☆
Aroma		☆ ☆ ☆ ☆ ☆
Body		☆ ☆ ☆ ☆ ☆
Taste		☆ ☆ ☆ ☆ ☆
Finish		☆ ☆ ☆ ☆ ☆

Tasting Notes	Temp & Brew time

Thoughts

Ratings ☆ ☆ ☆ ☆ ☆

Tea

Type _____ **Region** _____

Date _____

Appearance		☆ ☆ ☆ ☆ ☆
Aroma		☆ ☆ ☆ ☆ ☆
Body		☆ ☆ ☆ ☆ ☆
Taste		☆ ☆ ☆ ☆ ☆
Finish		☆ ☆ ☆ ☆ ☆

Tasting Notes	Temp & Brew time

Thoughts

Ratings ☆ ☆ ☆ ☆ ☆

Tea

Type _____   Region _____

Date _____

Appearance		☆ ☆ ☆ ☆ ☆
Aroma		☆ ☆ ☆ ☆ ☆
Body		☆ ☆ ☆ ☆ ☆
Taste		☆ ☆ ☆ ☆ ☆
Finish		☆ ☆ ☆ ☆ ☆

Tasting Notes	Temp & Brew time

Thoughts

Ratings ☆ ☆ ☆ ☆ ☆

Tea

Type _____   Region _____

Date _____

		Rating
Appearance		☆ ☆ ☆ ☆ ☆
Aroma		☆ ☆ ☆ ☆ ☆
Body		☆ ☆ ☆ ☆ ☆
Taste		☆ ☆ ☆ ☆ ☆
Finish		☆ ☆ ☆ ☆ ☆

Tasting Notes	Temp & Brew time

Thoughts

Ratings ☆ ☆ ☆ ☆ ☆

Tea

Type _____ Region _____

Date _____

Appearance		☆ ☆ ☆ ☆ ☆
Aroma		☆ ☆ ☆ ☆ ☆
Body		☆ ☆ ☆ ☆ ☆
Taste		☆ ☆ ☆ ☆ ☆
Finish		☆ ☆ ☆ ☆ ☆

Tasting Notes	Temp & Brew time

Thoughts

Ratings ☆ ☆ ☆ ☆ ☆

Tea

Type _____ Region _____

Date _____

Appearance		☆ ☆ ☆ ☆ ☆
Aroma		☆ ☆ ☆ ☆ ☆
Body		☆ ☆ ☆ ☆ ☆
Taste		☆ ☆ ☆ ☆ ☆
Finish		☆ ☆ ☆ ☆ ☆

Tasting Notes	Temp & Brew time

Thoughts

Ratings ☆ ☆ ☆ ☆ ☆

Tea

Type _____ Region _____

Date _____

Appearance		☆ ☆ ☆ ☆ ☆
Aroma		☆ ☆ ☆ ☆ ☆
Body		☆ ☆ ☆ ☆ ☆
Taste		☆ ☆ ☆ ☆ ☆
Finish		☆ ☆ ☆ ☆ ☆

Tasting Notes	Temp & Brew time

Thoughts

Ratings ☆ ☆ ☆ ☆ ☆

Tea

Type _____ **Region** _____

Date _____

Appearance		☆ ☆ ☆ ☆ ☆
Aroma		☆ ☆ ☆ ☆ ☆
Body		☆ ☆ ☆ ☆ ☆
Taste		☆ ☆ ☆ ☆ ☆
Finish		☆ ☆ ☆ ☆ ☆

Tasting Notes	Temp & Brew time

Thoughts

Ratings ☆ ☆ ☆ ☆ ☆

Tea

Type _____ Region _____

Date _____

Appearance		☆ ☆ ☆ ☆ ☆
Aroma		☆ ☆ ☆ ☆ ☆
Body		☆ ☆ ☆ ☆ ☆
Taste		☆ ☆ ☆ ☆ ☆
Finish		☆ ☆ ☆ ☆ ☆

Tasting Notes	Temp & Brew time

Thoughts

Ratings ☆ ☆ ☆ ☆ ☆

Tea

Type _____ Region _____

Date _____

Appearance		☆ ☆ ☆ ☆ ☆
Aroma		☆ ☆ ☆ ☆ ☆
Body		☆ ☆ ☆ ☆ ☆
Taste		☆ ☆ ☆ ☆ ☆
Finish		☆ ☆ ☆ ☆ ☆

Tasting Notes	Temp & Brew time

Thoughts

Ratings ☆ ☆ ☆ ☆ ☆

Tea

Type _____ Region _____

Date _____

Appearance		☆ ☆ ☆ ☆ ☆
Aroma		☆ ☆ ☆ ☆ ☆
Body		☆ ☆ ☆ ☆ ☆
Taste		☆ ☆ ☆ ☆ ☆
Finish		☆ ☆ ☆ ☆ ☆

Tasting Notes	Temp & Brew time

Thoughts

Ratings ☆ ☆ ☆ ☆ ☆

Tea _____

Type _____ Region _____

Date _____

Appearance		☆ ☆ ☆ ☆ ☆
Aroma		☆ ☆ ☆ ☆ ☆
Body		☆ ☆ ☆ ☆ ☆
Taste		☆ ☆ ☆ ☆ ☆
Finish		☆ ☆ ☆ ☆ ☆

Tasting Notes	Temp & Brew time

Thoughts

Ratings ☆ ☆ ☆ ☆ ☆

Tea

Type _____ Region _____

Date _____

Appearance		☆ ☆ ☆ ☆ ☆
Aroma		☆ ☆ ☆ ☆ ☆
Body		☆ ☆ ☆ ☆ ☆
Taste		☆ ☆ ☆ ☆ ☆
Finish		☆ ☆ ☆ ☆ ☆

Tasting Notes	Temp & Brew time

Thoughts

Ratings ☆ ☆ ☆ ☆ ☆

Tea _____

Type _____ Region _____

Date _____

Appearance		☆ ☆ ☆ ☆ ☆
Aroma		☆ ☆ ☆ ☆ ☆
Body		☆ ☆ ☆ ☆ ☆
Taste		☆ ☆ ☆ ☆ ☆
Finish		☆ ☆ ☆ ☆ ☆

Tasting Notes	Temp & Brew time

Thoughts

Ratings ☆ ☆ ☆ ☆ ☆

Tea

Type _____ Region _____

Date _____

Appearance		☆ ☆ ☆ ☆ ☆
Aroma		☆ ☆ ☆ ☆ ☆
Body		☆ ☆ ☆ ☆ ☆
Taste		☆ ☆ ☆ ☆ ☆
Finish		☆ ☆ ☆ ☆ ☆

Tasting Notes	Temp & Brew time

Thoughts

Ratings ☆ ☆ ☆ ☆ ☆

Tea _____

Type _____ Region _____

Date _____

Appearance		☆ ☆ ☆ ☆ ☆
Aroma		☆ ☆ ☆ ☆ ☆
Body		☆ ☆ ☆ ☆ ☆
Taste		☆ ☆ ☆ ☆ ☆
Finish		☆ ☆ ☆ ☆ ☆

Tasting Notes	Temp & Brew time

Thoughts

Ratings ☆ ☆ ☆ ☆ ☆

Tea

Type _____ Region _____

Date _____

Appearance		☆ ☆ ☆ ☆ ☆
Aroma		☆ ☆ ☆ ☆ ☆
Body		☆ ☆ ☆ ☆ ☆
Taste		☆ ☆ ☆ ☆ ☆
Finish		☆ ☆ ☆ ☆ ☆

Tasting Notes	Temp & Brew time

Thoughts

Ratings ☆ ☆ ☆ ☆ ☆

Tea _____

Type _____   Region _____

Date _____

Appearance		☆ ☆ ☆ ☆ ☆
Aroma		☆ ☆ ☆ ☆ ☆
Body		☆ ☆ ☆ ☆ ☆
Taste		☆ ☆ ☆ ☆ ☆
Finish		☆ ☆ ☆ ☆ ☆

Tasting Notes	Temp & Brew time

Thoughts

Ratings ☆ ☆ ☆ ☆ ☆

Tea

Type _____ Region _____

Date _____

Appearance		☆ ☆ ☆ ☆ ☆
Aroma		☆ ☆ ☆ ☆ ☆
Body		☆ ☆ ☆ ☆ ☆
Taste		☆ ☆ ☆ ☆ ☆
Finish		☆ ☆ ☆ ☆ ☆

Tasting Notes	Temp & Brew time

Thoughts

Ratings ☆ ☆ ☆ ☆ ☆

Tea

Type _____ Region _____

Date _____

Appearance		☆ ☆ ☆ ☆ ☆
Aroma		☆ ☆ ☆ ☆ ☆
Body		☆ ☆ ☆ ☆ ☆
Taste		☆ ☆ ☆ ☆ ☆
Finish		☆ ☆ ☆ ☆ ☆

Tasting Notes	Temp & Brew time

Thoughts

Ratings ☆ ☆ ☆ ☆ ☆

Tea

Type _____ Region _____

Date _____

Appearance		☆ ☆ ☆ ☆ ☆
Aroma		☆ ☆ ☆ ☆ ☆
Body		☆ ☆ ☆ ☆ ☆
Taste		☆ ☆ ☆ ☆ ☆
Finish		☆ ☆ ☆ ☆ ☆

Tasting Notes	Temp & Brew time

Thoughts

Ratings ☆ ☆ ☆ ☆ ☆

Tea

Type _____   **Region** _____

Date _____

Appearance		☆ ☆ ☆ ☆ ☆
Aroma		☆ ☆ ☆ ☆ ☆
Body		☆ ☆ ☆ ☆ ☆
Taste		☆ ☆ ☆ ☆ ☆
Finish		☆ ☆ ☆ ☆ ☆

Tasting Notes	Temp & Brew time

Thoughts

Ratings ☆ ☆ ☆ ☆ ☆

Tea

Type _____ Region _____

Date _____

Appearance		☆ ☆ ☆ ☆ ☆
Aroma		☆ ☆ ☆ ☆ ☆
Body		☆ ☆ ☆ ☆ ☆
Taste		☆ ☆ ☆ ☆ ☆
Finish		☆ ☆ ☆ ☆ ☆

Tasting Notes	Temp & Brew time

Thoughts

Ratings ☆ ☆ ☆ ☆ ☆

Tea

Type **_____** Region **_____**

Date **_____**

Appearance		☆ ☆ ☆ ☆ ☆
Aroma		☆ ☆ ☆ ☆ ☆
Body		☆ ☆ ☆ ☆ ☆
Taste		☆ ☆ ☆ ☆ ☆
Finish		☆ ☆ ☆ ☆ ☆

Tasting Notes	Temp & Brew time

Thoughts

Ratings ☆ ☆ ☆ ☆ ☆

Tea

Type _____ Region _____

Date _____

Appearance		☆ ☆ ☆ ☆ ☆
Aroma		☆ ☆ ☆ ☆ ☆
Body		☆ ☆ ☆ ☆ ☆
Taste		☆ ☆ ☆ ☆ ☆
Finish		☆ ☆ ☆ ☆ ☆

Tasting Notes	Temp & Brew time

Thoughts

Ratings ☆ ☆ ☆ ☆ ☆

Tea

Type _____ Region _____

Date _____

Appearance		☆ ☆ ☆ ☆ ☆
Aroma		☆ ☆ ☆ ☆ ☆
Body		☆ ☆ ☆ ☆ ☆
Taste		☆ ☆ ☆ ☆ ☆
Finish		☆ ☆ ☆ ☆ ☆

Tasting Notes	Temp & Brew time

Thoughts

Ratings ☆ ☆ ☆ ☆ ☆

Tea

Type _____ Region _____

Date _____

Appearance		☆ ☆ ☆ ☆ ☆
Aroma		☆ ☆ ☆ ☆ ☆
Body		☆ ☆ ☆ ☆ ☆
Taste		☆ ☆ ☆ ☆ ☆
Finish		☆ ☆ ☆ ☆ ☆

Tasting Notes	Temp & Brew time

Thoughts

Ratings ☆ ☆ ☆ ☆ ☆

Tea

Type _____   Region _____

Date _____

		Rating
Appearance		☆ ☆ ☆ ☆ ☆
Aroma		☆ ☆ ☆ ☆ ☆
Body		☆ ☆ ☆ ☆ ☆
Taste		☆ ☆ ☆ ☆ ☆
Finish		☆ ☆ ☆ ☆ ☆

Tasting Notes	Temp & Brew time

Thoughts

Ratings ☆ ☆ ☆ ☆ ☆

Tea

Type _____ Region _____

Date _____

Appearance		☆ ☆ ☆ ☆ ☆
Aroma		☆ ☆ ☆ ☆ ☆
Body		☆ ☆ ☆ ☆ ☆
Taste		☆ ☆ ☆ ☆ ☆
Finish		☆ ☆ ☆ ☆ ☆

Tasting Notes	Temp & Brew time

Thoughts

Ratings ☆ ☆ ☆ ☆ ☆

Tea

Type _____ Region _____

Date _____

Appearance		☆ ☆ ☆ ☆ ☆
Aroma		☆ ☆ ☆ ☆ ☆
Body		☆ ☆ ☆ ☆ ☆
Taste		☆ ☆ ☆ ☆ ☆
Finish		☆ ☆ ☆ ☆ ☆

Tasting Notes	Temp & Brew time

Thoughts

Ratings ☆ ☆ ☆ ☆ ☆

Tea

Type _____ Region _____

Date _____

Appearance		☆ ☆ ☆ ☆ ☆
Aroma		☆ ☆ ☆ ☆ ☆
Body		☆ ☆ ☆ ☆ ☆
Taste		☆ ☆ ☆ ☆ ☆
Finish		☆ ☆ ☆ ☆ ☆

Tasting Notes	Temp & Brew time

Thoughts

Ratings ☆ ☆ ☆ ☆ ☆

Tea

Type _____   **Region** _____

Date _____

Appearance		☆ ☆ ☆ ☆ ☆
Aroma		☆ ☆ ☆ ☆ ☆
Body		☆ ☆ ☆ ☆ ☆
Taste		☆ ☆ ☆ ☆ ☆
Finish		☆ ☆ ☆ ☆ ☆

Tasting Notes	Temp & Brew time

Thoughts

Ratings ☆ ☆ ☆ ☆ ☆

Tea

Type _____ Region _____

Date _____

Appearance		☆ ☆ ☆ ☆ ☆
Aroma		☆ ☆ ☆ ☆ ☆
Body		☆ ☆ ☆ ☆ ☆
Taste		☆ ☆ ☆ ☆ ☆
Finish		☆ ☆ ☆ ☆ ☆

Tasting Notes	Temp & Brew time

Thoughts

Ratings ☆ ☆ ☆ ☆ ☆

Tea

Type _____ Region _____

Date _____

Appearance		☆ ☆ ☆ ☆ ☆
Aroma		☆ ☆ ☆ ☆ ☆
Body		☆ ☆ ☆ ☆ ☆
Taste		☆ ☆ ☆ ☆ ☆
Finish		☆ ☆ ☆ ☆ ☆

Tasting Notes	Temp & Brew time

Thoughts

Ratings ☆ ☆ ☆ ☆ ☆

Tea

Type _____ **Region** _____

Date _____

Appearance		☆ ☆ ☆ ☆ ☆
Aroma		☆ ☆ ☆ ☆ ☆
Body		☆ ☆ ☆ ☆ ☆
Taste		☆ ☆ ☆ ☆ ☆
Finish		☆ ☆ ☆ ☆ ☆

Tasting Notes	Temp & Brew time

Thoughts

Ratings ☆ ☆ ☆ ☆ ☆

Tea

Type _____ Region _____

Date _____

Appearance		☆ ☆ ☆ ☆ ☆
Aroma		☆ ☆ ☆ ☆ ☆
Body		☆ ☆ ☆ ☆ ☆
Taste		☆ ☆ ☆ ☆ ☆
Finish		☆ ☆ ☆ ☆ ☆

Tasting Notes	Temp & Brew time

Thoughts

Ratings ☆ ☆ ☆ ☆ ☆

Tea

Type _____ Region _____

Date _____

Appearance		☆ ☆ ☆ ☆ ☆
Aroma		☆ ☆ ☆ ☆ ☆
Body		☆ ☆ ☆ ☆ ☆
Taste		☆ ☆ ☆ ☆ ☆
Finish		☆ ☆ ☆ ☆ ☆

Tasting Notes	Temp & Brew time

Thoughts

Ratings ☆ ☆ ☆ ☆ ☆

Tea

Type _____ **Region** _____

Date _____

Appearance		☆ ☆ ☆ ☆ ☆
Aroma		☆ ☆ ☆ ☆ ☆
Body		☆ ☆ ☆ ☆ ☆
Taste		☆ ☆ ☆ ☆ ☆
Finish		☆ ☆ ☆ ☆ ☆

Tasting Notes	Temp & Brew time

Thoughts

Ratings ☆ ☆ ☆ ☆ ☆

Tea

Type _____ Region _____

Date _____

Appearance		☆ ☆ ☆ ☆ ☆
Aroma		☆ ☆ ☆ ☆ ☆
Body		☆ ☆ ☆ ☆ ☆
Taste		☆ ☆ ☆ ☆ ☆
Finish		☆ ☆ ☆ ☆ ☆

Tasting Notes	Temp & Brew time

Thoughts

Ratings ☆ ☆ ☆ ☆ ☆

Tea

Type _____   **Region** _____

Date _____

Appearance		☆ ☆ ☆ ☆ ☆
Aroma		☆ ☆ ☆ ☆ ☆
Body		☆ ☆ ☆ ☆ ☆
Taste		☆ ☆ ☆ ☆ ☆
Finish		☆ ☆ ☆ ☆ ☆

Tasting Notes	Temp & Brew time

Thoughts

Ratings ☆ ☆ ☆ ☆ ☆

Tea

Type _____ Region _____

Date _____

Appearance		☆ ☆ ☆ ☆ ☆
Aroma		☆ ☆ ☆ ☆ ☆
Body		☆ ☆ ☆ ☆ ☆
Taste		☆ ☆ ☆ ☆ ☆
Finish		☆ ☆ ☆ ☆ ☆

Tasting Notes	Temp & Brew time

Thoughts

Ratings ☆ ☆ ☆ ☆ ☆

Tea

Type _____ **Region** _____

Date _____

Appearance		☆ ☆ ☆ ☆ ☆
Aroma		☆ ☆ ☆ ☆ ☆
Body		☆ ☆ ☆ ☆ ☆
Taste		☆ ☆ ☆ ☆ ☆
Finish		☆ ☆ ☆ ☆ ☆

Tasting Notes	Temp & Brew time

Thoughts

Ratings ☆ ☆ ☆ ☆ ☆

Tea

Type _____ Region _____

Date _____

Appearance		☆ ☆ ☆ ☆ ☆
Aroma		☆ ☆ ☆ ☆ ☆
Body		☆ ☆ ☆ ☆ ☆
Taste		☆ ☆ ☆ ☆ ☆
Finish		☆ ☆ ☆ ☆ ☆

Tasting Notes	Temp & Brew time

Thoughts

Ratings ☆ ☆ ☆ ☆ ☆

Tea _____

Type _____ Region _____

Date _____

Appearance		☆ ☆ ☆ ☆ ☆
Aroma		☆ ☆ ☆ ☆ ☆
Body		☆ ☆ ☆ ☆ ☆
Taste		☆ ☆ ☆ ☆ ☆
Finish		☆ ☆ ☆ ☆ ☆

Tasting Notes	Temp & Brew time

Thoughts

Ratings ☆ ☆ ☆ ☆ ☆

Tea _____

Type _____ Region _____

Date _____

Appearance		☆ ☆ ☆ ☆ ☆
Aroma		☆ ☆ ☆ ☆ ☆
Body		☆ ☆ ☆ ☆ ☆
Taste		☆ ☆ ☆ ☆ ☆
Finish		☆ ☆ ☆ ☆ ☆

Tasting Notes	Temp & Brew time

Thoughts

Ratings ☆ ☆ ☆ ☆ ☆

Tea

Type _____ Region _____

Date _____

Appearance		☆ ☆ ☆ ☆ ☆
Aroma		☆ ☆ ☆ ☆ ☆
Body		☆ ☆ ☆ ☆ ☆
Taste		☆ ☆ ☆ ☆ ☆
Finish		☆ ☆ ☆ ☆ ☆

Tasting Notes	Temp & Brew time

Thoughts

Ratings ☆ ☆ ☆ ☆ ☆

Tea

Type _____ Region _____

Date _____

Appearance		☆ ☆ ☆ ☆ ☆
Aroma		☆ ☆ ☆ ☆ ☆
Body		☆ ☆ ☆ ☆ ☆
Taste		☆ ☆ ☆ ☆ ☆
Finish		☆ ☆ ☆ ☆ ☆

Tasting Notes	Temp & Brew time

Thoughts

Ratings ☆ ☆ ☆ ☆ ☆

Tea

Type _____   **Region** _____

Date _____

Appearance		☆ ☆ ☆ ☆ ☆
Aroma		☆ ☆ ☆ ☆ ☆
Body		☆ ☆ ☆ ☆ ☆
Taste		☆ ☆ ☆ ☆ ☆
Finish		☆ ☆ ☆ ☆ ☆

Tasting Notes	Temp & Brew time

Thoughts

Ratings ☆ ☆ ☆ ☆ ☆

Tea _____

Type _____ Region _____

Date _____

Appearance		☆ ☆ ☆ ☆ ☆
Aroma		☆ ☆ ☆ ☆ ☆
Body		☆ ☆ ☆ ☆ ☆
Taste		☆ ☆ ☆ ☆ ☆
Finish		☆ ☆ ☆ ☆ ☆

Tasting Notes	Temp & Brew time

Thoughts

Ratings ☆ ☆ ☆ ☆ ☆

Tea

Type _____ **Region** _____

Date _____

Appearance		☆ ☆ ☆ ☆ ☆
Aroma		☆ ☆ ☆ ☆ ☆
Body		☆ ☆ ☆ ☆ ☆
Taste		☆ ☆ ☆ ☆ ☆
Finish		☆ ☆ ☆ ☆ ☆

Tasting Notes	Temp & Brew time

Thoughts

Ratings ☆ ☆ ☆ ☆ ☆

Tea

Type _____ **Region** _____

Date _____

Appearance		☆ ☆ ☆ ☆ ☆
Aroma		☆ ☆ ☆ ☆ ☆
Body		☆ ☆ ☆ ☆ ☆
Taste		☆ ☆ ☆ ☆ ☆
Finish		☆ ☆ ☆ ☆ ☆

Tasting Notes	Temp & Brew time

Thoughts

Ratings ☆ ☆ ☆ ☆ ☆

Tea

Type _____ Region _____

Date _____

Appearance		☆ ☆ ☆ ☆ ☆
Aroma		☆ ☆ ☆ ☆ ☆
Body		☆ ☆ ☆ ☆ ☆
Taste		☆ ☆ ☆ ☆ ☆
Finish		☆ ☆ ☆ ☆ ☆

Tasting Notes	Temp & Brew time

Thoughts

Ratings ☆ ☆ ☆ ☆ ☆

Tea

Type _____ Region _____

Date _____

Appearance		☆ ☆ ☆ ☆ ☆
Aroma		☆ ☆ ☆ ☆ ☆
Body		☆ ☆ ☆ ☆ ☆
Taste		☆ ☆ ☆ ☆ ☆
Finish		☆ ☆ ☆ ☆ ☆

Tasting Notes	Temp & Brew time

Thoughts

Ratings ☆ ☆ ☆ ☆ ☆

Tea _____

Type _____ Region _____

Date _____

Appearance		☆ ☆ ☆ ☆ ☆
Aroma		☆ ☆ ☆ ☆ ☆
Body		☆ ☆ ☆ ☆ ☆
Taste		☆ ☆ ☆ ☆ ☆
Finish		☆ ☆ ☆ ☆ ☆

Tasting Notes	Temp & Brew time

Thoughts

Ratings ☆ ☆ ☆ ☆ ☆

Tea

Type _____ Region _____

Date _____

Appearance		☆ ☆ ☆ ☆ ☆
Aroma		☆ ☆ ☆ ☆ ☆
Body		☆ ☆ ☆ ☆ ☆
Taste		☆ ☆ ☆ ☆ ☆
Finish		☆ ☆ ☆ ☆ ☆

Tasting Notes	Temp & Brew time

Thoughts

Ratings ☆ ☆ ☆ ☆ ☆

Tea

Type _____ Region _____

Date _____

Appearance		☆ ☆ ☆ ☆ ☆
Aroma		☆ ☆ ☆ ☆ ☆
Body		☆ ☆ ☆ ☆ ☆
Taste		☆ ☆ ☆ ☆ ☆
Finish		☆ ☆ ☆ ☆ ☆

Tasting Notes	Temp & Brew time

Thoughts

Ratings ☆ ☆ ☆ ☆ ☆

Tea

Type _____ Region _____

Date _____

Appearance		☆ ☆ ☆ ☆ ☆
Aroma		☆ ☆ ☆ ☆ ☆
Body		☆ ☆ ☆ ☆ ☆
Taste		☆ ☆ ☆ ☆ ☆
Finish		☆ ☆ ☆ ☆ ☆

Tasting Notes	Temp & Brew time

Thoughts

Ratings ☆ ☆ ☆ ☆ ☆

Tea

Type _____ **Region** _____

Date _____

Appearance		☆ ☆ ☆ ☆ ☆
Aroma		☆ ☆ ☆ ☆ ☆
Body		☆ ☆ ☆ ☆ ☆
Taste		☆ ☆ ☆ ☆ ☆
Finish		☆ ☆ ☆ ☆ ☆

Tasting Notes	Temp & Brew time

Thoughts

Ratings ☆ ☆ ☆ ☆ ☆

Tea

Type _____ **Region** _____

Date _____

Appearance		☆ ☆ ☆ ☆ ☆
Aroma		☆ ☆ ☆ ☆ ☆
Body		☆ ☆ ☆ ☆ ☆
Taste		☆ ☆ ☆ ☆ ☆
Finish		☆ ☆ ☆ ☆ ☆

Tasting Notes	Temp & Brew time

Thoughts

Ratings ☆ ☆ ☆ ☆ ☆

Tea _____

Type _____ Region _____

Date _____

Appearance		☆ ☆ ☆ ☆ ☆
Aroma		☆ ☆ ☆ ☆ ☆
Body		☆ ☆ ☆ ☆ ☆
Taste		☆ ☆ ☆ ☆ ☆
Finish		☆ ☆ ☆ ☆ ☆

Tasting Notes	Temp & Brew time

Thoughts

Ratings ☆ ☆ ☆ ☆ ☆

Tea

Type _____ **Region** _____

Date _____

Appearance		☆ ☆ ☆ ☆ ☆
Aroma		☆ ☆ ☆ ☆ ☆
Body		☆ ☆ ☆ ☆ ☆
Taste		☆ ☆ ☆ ☆ ☆
Finish		☆ ☆ ☆ ☆ ☆

Tasting Notes	Temp & Brew time

Thoughts

Ratings ☆ ☆ ☆ ☆ ☆

Tea

Type _____ Region _____

Date _____

Appearance		☆ ☆ ☆ ☆ ☆
Aroma		☆ ☆ ☆ ☆ ☆
Body		☆ ☆ ☆ ☆ ☆
Taste		☆ ☆ ☆ ☆ ☆
Finish		☆ ☆ ☆ ☆ ☆

Tasting Notes	Temp & Brew time

Thoughts

Ratings ☆ ☆ ☆ ☆ ☆

Tea

Type _____ **Region** _____

Date _____

Appearance		☆ ☆ ☆ ☆ ☆
Aroma		☆ ☆ ☆ ☆ ☆
Body		☆ ☆ ☆ ☆ ☆
Taste		☆ ☆ ☆ ☆ ☆
Finish		☆ ☆ ☆ ☆ ☆

Tasting Notes	Temp & Brew time

Thoughts

Ratings ☆ ☆ ☆ ☆ ☆

Tea

Type _____ **Region** _____

Date _____

Appearance		☆ ☆ ☆ ☆ ☆
Aroma		☆ ☆ ☆ ☆ ☆
Body		☆ ☆ ☆ ☆ ☆
Taste		☆ ☆ ☆ ☆ ☆
Finish		☆ ☆ ☆ ☆ ☆

Tasting Notes	Temp & Brew time

Thoughts

Ratings ☆ ☆ ☆ ☆ ☆

Tea

Type _____ Region _____

Date _____

Appearance		☆ ☆ ☆ ☆ ☆
Aroma		☆ ☆ ☆ ☆ ☆
Body		☆ ☆ ☆ ☆ ☆
Taste		☆ ☆ ☆ ☆ ☆
Finish		☆ ☆ ☆ ☆ ☆

Tasting Notes	Temp & Brew time

Thoughts

Ratings ☆ ☆ ☆ ☆ ☆

Tea

Type _____ **Region** _____

Date _____

Appearance		☆ ☆ ☆ ☆ ☆
Aroma		☆ ☆ ☆ ☆ ☆
Body		☆ ☆ ☆ ☆ ☆
Taste		☆ ☆ ☆ ☆ ☆
Finish		☆ ☆ ☆ ☆ ☆

Tasting Notes	Temp & Brew time

Thoughts

Ratings ☆ ☆ ☆ ☆ ☆

Tea

Type _____ Region _____

Date _____

Appearance		☆ ☆ ☆ ☆ ☆
Aroma		☆ ☆ ☆ ☆ ☆
Body		☆ ☆ ☆ ☆ ☆
Taste		☆ ☆ ☆ ☆ ☆
Finish		☆ ☆ ☆ ☆ ☆

Tasting Notes	Temp & Brew time

Thoughts

Ratings ☆ ☆ ☆ ☆ ☆

Tea

Type _____ **Region** _____

Date _____

Appearance		☆ ☆ ☆ ☆ ☆
Aroma		☆ ☆ ☆ ☆ ☆
Body		☆ ☆ ☆ ☆ ☆
Taste		☆ ☆ ☆ ☆ ☆
Finish		☆ ☆ ☆ ☆ ☆

Tasting Notes	Temp & Brew time

Thoughts

Ratings ☆ ☆ ☆ ☆ ☆

Tea

Type _____ Region _____

Date _____

Appearance		☆ ☆ ☆ ☆ ☆
Aroma		☆ ☆ ☆ ☆ ☆
Body		☆ ☆ ☆ ☆ ☆
Taste		☆ ☆ ☆ ☆ ☆
Finish		☆ ☆ ☆ ☆ ☆

Tasting Notes	Temp & Brew time

Thoughts

Ratings ☆ ☆ ☆ ☆ ☆

Tea

Type _____ Region _____

Date _____

Appearance		☆ ☆ ☆ ☆ ☆
Aroma		☆ ☆ ☆ ☆ ☆
Body		☆ ☆ ☆ ☆ ☆
Taste		☆ ☆ ☆ ☆ ☆
Finish		☆ ☆ ☆ ☆ ☆

Tasting Notes	Temp & Brew time

Thoughts

Ratings ☆ ☆ ☆ ☆ ☆

Tea

Type _____ Region _____

Date _____

Appearance		☆ ☆ ☆ ☆ ☆
Aroma		☆ ☆ ☆ ☆ ☆
Body		☆ ☆ ☆ ☆ ☆
Taste		☆ ☆ ☆ ☆ ☆
Finish		☆ ☆ ☆ ☆ ☆

Tasting Notes	Temp & Brew time

Thoughts

Ratings ☆ ☆ ☆ ☆ ☆

Tea

Type _____ Region _____

Date _____

Appearance		☆ ☆ ☆ ☆ ☆
Aroma		☆ ☆ ☆ ☆ ☆
Body		☆ ☆ ☆ ☆ ☆
Taste		☆ ☆ ☆ ☆ ☆
Finish		☆ ☆ ☆ ☆ ☆

Tasting Notes	Temp & Brew time

Thoughts

Ratings ☆ ☆ ☆ ☆ ☆

Tea

Type _____ **Region** _____

Date _____

Appearance		☆ ☆ ☆ ☆ ☆
Aroma		☆ ☆ ☆ ☆ ☆
Body		☆ ☆ ☆ ☆ ☆
Taste		☆ ☆ ☆ ☆ ☆
Finish		☆ ☆ ☆ ☆ ☆

Tasting Notes	Temp & Brew time

Thoughts

Ratings ☆ ☆ ☆ ☆ ☆

Tea

Type _____ Region _____

Date _____

Appearance		☆ ☆ ☆ ☆ ☆
Aroma		☆ ☆ ☆ ☆ ☆
Body		☆ ☆ ☆ ☆ ☆
Taste		☆ ☆ ☆ ☆ ☆
Finish		☆ ☆ ☆ ☆ ☆

Tasting Notes	Temp & Brew time

Thoughts

Ratings ☆ ☆ ☆ ☆ ☆

Tea

Type _____ Region _____

Date _____

Appearance		☆ ☆ ☆ ☆ ☆
Aroma		☆ ☆ ☆ ☆ ☆
Body		☆ ☆ ☆ ☆ ☆
Taste		☆ ☆ ☆ ☆ ☆
Finish		☆ ☆ ☆ ☆ ☆

Tasting Notes	Temp & Brew time

Thoughts

Ratings ☆ ☆ ☆ ☆ ☆

www.ingramcontent.com/pod-product-compliance
Lightning Source LLC
Chambersburg PA
CBHW072105280526
45788CB00006B/2405